Survival Guide for Children:

30 Important Lessons For Your Kids to Be Protected in Any Situation

Table of Contents

Introduction

In this world we live in, it seems you have two kinds of parents. You have those who are always over their children's shoulders, looking at what they are doing, and wrapping bubble wrap around their every move.

Then, you have those parents who don't seem to be at all concerned with what their child is doing, nor do they seem to even notice when their child is doing something that you consider very dangerous.

Every parent is different, and each parent has their own style when it comes to the safety of their children. But, there is one common thing that ties all parents together, and that's the fact they want their kids to be safe and happy.

But there are times when you aren't going to be around, and there are times when your child has to know how to handle a situation themselves. You see, in the world we live in, though you may do your best to ensure that all is perfect, you have to also make sure your child knows what to do when things aren't perfect.

It's never fun to think about the things that could happen, but the fact of the matter is that there are bad things that do happen, and you want your child to know what to do when they do. Whether you run errands and your child wanders off, or if you are out for a few minutes and a stranger comes to the door, you have to make sure your child is prepared.

But how do you know what to say? How do you teach your child to be prepared for something that without making them fear all of the other things in life that could go wrong? You want to reassure your child that things are going to be ok, but you also want him to be able to handle anything that could go wrong.

This book is the book for you. In it, I am going to show you everything you need to know to teach your child how to behave in a variety of situations, and build the confidence they need to pull through. A little bit of confidence can go a long way, and with this book, you can instill all the confidence your child needs.

Practice the scenarios so your child is familiar with how to act, and review what you have taught your child every now and then. You don't want to be paranoid, and you don't want your child to be scared of the things in life, but you do want your child to be ready.

And with this book, you can rest assured knowing your child is ready for anything, and can handle any situation that arises. Take the confidence you have in your child's abilities and build up their confidence in themselves, and you will be ready for anything.

Now let's get started.

Chapter 1 – Safety Starts at Home

We all do everything we can to ensure that our homes are safety zones for our families. Whether it's child-proofing every room in the house to taking down anything and everything your child might find frightening, you are there to protect them from anything and everything.

But there are times you may not be there directly, and your child is going to need to know what to do. By giving your child a game plan, you are giving them the tools they need to make it through any situation quickly and easily. This is going to provide peace of mind to you and your child both.

Here are a few situations you hope will never happen, but you want to make sure your child is ready for them in the event they do. Start the conversation by asking your child what would they do if __________________ then give them the answer for each situation.

If you are home and:

A stranger comes to the door

First of all, whatever the reason your child is home alone, make sure they know to lock the doors. Lock any and all doors and keep them locked until your return.

If you are home, teach your child to respond the same way.

Never go to the door or open the door. Don't look out through windows or try to talk to the stranger. If you're home, teach your child to come get you. If you are not, teach your child to stay away from the door and call you.

You can't find your kitty or puppy

Some houses are large, and some animals are good at hiding. If your child can't find his pet, teach him to come to you about it first. Never, ever go outside searching for the pet, or try to get into dangerous areas in the house.

Come to you first, and you'll look for the pet together.

There's a fire or other safety hazard

Whether it's something burning on the stove, a candle, or anything else, teach your child what to do with fire. If your child is old enough, show him how to use the extinguisher.

Teach him how to get out of the house and go to the safety zone if the house is on fire, and teach him to feel doorknobs first to see if there's fire in the room before he opens the door.

And, of course, teach him how to call 911 and what to say on the phone when he does.

Your mom or dad is stuck in a room and you can't get them out

Locks get jammed and doors get stuck, especially in older houses. Teach your child what to do if you are locked in a room in your home and can't get out. Teach him who to call and what to say, and make sure the phone is where he can safely and easily reach.

Something happens to your mom or dad and there's no one else home

Again, things happen. Whether it's an unforeseen health issue or another kind of emergency, make sure your child knows who to call and what to do if he is suddenly faced with something happening to you.

Teaching your child to remain calm in the situation as well as what to do is going to make it a lot easier for both of you if it ever happens.

Chapter 2 – At School and at Play

As much as you would like to be, you can't be there for your child all the time, every day. It's important that your child knows what to do when he's away from you, and how to handle a variety of situations that may arise.

Teach your child how to remain calm and handle the things that could happen, and your child isn't going to bat an eye if they ever do. Approach this topic the same as you did with safety in the house. Simply ask your child what they would do, and give them the right answer.

Practice until you are certain your child knows what to do.

When you are playing with friends or at school and:

Someone gets hurt badly

Teach your child how to handle the injury, depending on what it is. If another child hits his head or breaks his arm, it's going to be handled differently than if he were to get cut.

Teach your child who to get a hold of and how, and what to do for the injury itself.

A stranger tries to give you something

It doesn't matter what it is or what they say, make sure your child knows to never, ever take anything... anything... from strangers. Teach him to also get away from the stranger and find a trusted adult to tell what happened.

A stranger asks for your help

Again, teach your child that under no circumstances can he or she help strangers. Tell your child that strangers don't ask children for help, and to never do anything the stranger asks, no matter how harmless it seems. Teach him to also get away from the stranger and find a trusted adult to tell what happened.

A stranger asks if you will go with them

Teach your child that under no circumstances can he or she go with strangers. Tell your child that strangers don't ask children for help, and to never do anything the stranger asks, no matter how harmless it seems.

Even if the stranger asks if your child will just look around the area with them, teach your child to never do it.

Teach him to also get away from the stranger and find a trusted adult to tell what happened.

Your friend wants you to do something you know you're not supposed to do

Friends may have the best intentions, and they may not mean any harm by the things they do, but when it comes to the rules you have made, teach your child to stick with these rules no matter what.

Let your child know that families are different, and let him know that just because his friend can do something, it doesn't mean he's allowed to. Teach your child how to nicely tell his friend no, and stay firm on his choice, regardless of what his friend says or does.

If necessary, teach your child to get another adult involved with the situation.

Chapter 3 – Lessons for Around Town

Running errands and getting a few things done around town isn't a big deal, unless your child doesn't know what to do in different situations. You never want to think about your child getting lost, and you certainly don't want to think of anything bad happening, but it's important that you teach your child what to do in a variety of situations.

Use the same teaching method as you do with other situations, asking your child what he would do, and give him the answer.

If you are out running errands with your mom or dad and:

You get lost

Teach your child to go to the front of the store and ask a cashier to call for you. Teach your child to also never go to any stranger in the store, only someone who works for the store.

Teach your child how to know how is working for the store, and where to go if they ever need to. Teach your child to remain calm in the situation, and practice until he's comfortable doing it.

You get stuck in a room

Bathrooms and dressing rooms can have tight locks, and your child is going to need to know what to do if he gets stuck. Tell him how to attract the attention of an employee, and how to find you if this happens.

If your child has a cell phone, show him how to call you and tell you what is going on.

You're in a car and it's too hot

Even if you run into a store for only a second, it can get hot in a car. It's important that your child knows what to do if he is feeling too hot. Open windows, or, if necessary, open a door.

Make sure your child understands the importance of not overheating, and that no matter what they can get out of there if they need to.

A strange dog runs up to you

Whether the dog is with its owner or on its own, it's very important that you teach your child how to handle it if this situation arises. Stay away from the dog until you have permission to pet it, and if the dog is alone, back away from it and shout at it to leave.

Never approach a strange dog, and stay away from any that run up to you.

Your own dog or cat runs away

If your child's pet runs away, it's really hard for them to understand what is happening, but it's really important that your child also understands not chasing after the animal.

Your child could run into the street and get hit by a car. Your child could get lost themselves, or any number of other things could happen. Teach your child to remain calm and get you if something like this happens, and what to do if they see their pet run away.

Make sure they know that you will handle it, and they shouldn't chase after the animal themselves.

Chapter 4 – Things to Know When You Stay the Night

We all want to be with our children as much as possible. To be able to watch them and ensure they are safe and making the right choices, to keep an eye on them and watch out for things that could go wrong, and to just be there if they have any needs at all.

But, as your kids begin to grow up, they also begin to want to do things without you there. As you well know, this means they are going to be at a friend's house spending the night or going other places without you there to supervise.

The more this happens, the more you want to know without a doubt they are able to handle things themselves.

But, it can be hard to know what to say when you prepare your child to spend the night away from you. This is especially true if you don't want them to think you don't like the way their friend does things at their house.

But, as with the other lessons you have been teaching your child, the best thing to do is to just approach it as you did the other topics. Ask your child first what they would do in that situation, then tell them what the right answer is.

When you stay over at a friend's house for the night you must know what to do if:

Something happens that wasn't part of the plan

Now, this doesn't have to be a bad thing, and you can let your child know this. If they are supposed to be at their friend's house, and they decide to leave the house for any reason, make sure your child knows if they ought to call you or not.

If something comes up and they can no longer spend the night, let them know they are supposed to call you, and if their friend decides they are going to do something which is normally against the rules for your child to do, let them know how to handle that situation as well.

You want your child to have the confidence to do what they know is right in any situation, but part of building this confidence is by letting them know the right course of action for anything that could come up.

The key is to emphasize to your child that they aren't doing anything wrong when they do what you instruct them to do, regardless of what the other child is allowed to do.

For example:

Your child is at his friend Bobby's house, and Bobby is allowed to go to the skate park unsupervised. You prefer that there is an adult present when your child goes, and you let your child know this.

When he's at Bobby's house, Bobby decides they ought to go skating together. While this isn't anything bad, you need to instruct your child to always stand firm in what he is allowed to do, and call you to either get permission to do something else, or to come pick him up.

Make sure your child knows there's nothing to be upset about, and that he's doing the right thing.

An emergency happens at your friend's house

Things happen, and can happen, anywhere. No matter where your child goes, you want him to be prepared and know what to do, so it's important to prepare him for possible emergencies, even at a friend's house.

Make sure he knows your number and how to call 911, and that he remains calm enough to do that if the need ever arises.

The power goes out

The power going out can be scary enough for a small child when he's at your house, but it can be even harder when he's at someone else's. Teach your child how to handle a power outage without being scared, and to call you if there's ever a reason.

It's a good idea for your child to have their own phone when they are away from the house... this is going to give them instant access to you whenever they need to or wherever they are.

You lost or broke your phone and can't reach your parents

Teach your child what your phone number is, and where to find a phone to call you from in the event his phone is missing.

You may find it incredibly convenient to put your phone number in your child's phone, but for as nice as that is, you must also make sure your child knows what your phone number is.

Phones can get lost, broken, stolen, or forgotten, and if your child doesn't know what your phone number is, there's no way for him to be able to reach you from any other phone. Post your phone number somewhere that is easily accessible anyway, then help your child memorize your number.

Practice to make sure he knows for sure what it is, and rest assured your child knows how to get a hold of you whenever he needs.

You decide you want to leave for any reason

Things happen, and sometimes your child just decides he doesn't want to stay the night after all. It's up to you to teach your child that it's ok to change his mind, and to simply call you or ask his friend's parent to drop him off back at home if it does.

Some children feel embarrassed, or put themselves in uncomfortable situations merely because they don't know how to handle it if they don't. Make sure your child knows it's ok to change his mind, and that you're going to be there to get him if he does.

Chapter 5 – Important Lessons for Travel

Travel is one of the most stressful things you have to deal with when it comes to your family, whether you are going on a trip together or not. Perhaps your child is going on some sort of field trip, or maybe there's a family vacation coming up. With all the excitement there's still a mix of worry, and you need to make sure you are completely certain your child is going to be ready for the adventure.

Ask your child what he would do in these situations, just as you do with all other situations. Listen to how they would handle things, and why, then teach them what the right thing to do is.

Practice with your children to ensure they fully understand what to do, and rest assured they'll be just fine on the next trip, no matter what happens.

Whether you and your family are on vacation or if you are on a trip with school, it's important to know what to do if:

You get lost or separated from the group

Teach your child the best thing to do is find a common area and ask for help. Don't ask random strangers for help, but rather, ask an employee.

For example, if the class is on a school trip and your child gets separated from the group, instruct them to go into the nearest store and inform the person behind the counter of what happened. Make sure they know to include their name and what school they are from, and where they were supposed to be going.

When you child knows the proper information to relay, they are able to get the help they need quickly.

You miss the stop you were supposed to get off at

Things happen, and if your child happens to fall asleep on the bus or not be paying attention and get off when they should, they may miss their stop. This could cause them to panic and frantically search for help.

Teach your child to inform the bus driver of what happened, and who to call. He will know to call you in the event that ever happens and let you know where he is, as well as have the bus driver's help to get back where he needs to go.

You can't find your money

Teach your child what you want him to do if he is ever on a trip and can't find his money, ticket, or anything else he was supposed to have with him. Teach him that panicking is never the right answer, and can only make matters worse. Teach him to inform the teacher or whoever is in charge of what happened, and let him know that it's all going to be ok.

For a child, many things that may not seem like too big a deal to us are incredibly scary to them. Teach your child to be calm in all situations, and rest assured he's going to stay calm when he needs to.

It's too hot or cold outside

You never know the kind of weather you will run into when you are on a trip, and you never know how your child is going to react. Teach your child to pay attention to the weather, and if he sees things changing, to act accordingly.

You may not always be there to tell your child to put on a jacket, or to bring a jacket with him when he's outside, but you can teach him to pay attention to the weather and prepare for things himself.

The more prepared he is, the better he's going to handle any situation.

You feel sick

There are a number of contributing factors that can make your child feel suddenly ill, even if they were perfectly fine when they left.

Teach your child what phone numbers he needs to know and who to tell if he suddenly feels sick, and let him know that it will be taken care of. Many children will stay quiet even though they feel ill simply because they aren't sure how to handle the situation.

Teach your child to speak up when he feels sick, and to speak up right away. Make sure he knows it's ok and that everything is going to be taken care of.

Chapter 6 – Anytime, Anywhere Lessons

Sometimes it doesn't matter where you are, and sometimes it doesn't matter what you are doing. There are times when you just simply need to be prepared for whatever happens, and prepare your children for the unexpected.

In this last chapter, I want to address the things to teach your children when there are no particular circumstances going on. These are the things you have to watch out for just in case they happen, and things you will feel better knowing your children are aware of.

Sometimes it doesn't matter where you are, there are still things you need to know. What would you do if:

You or your friend has accidentally swallowed poison of some kind

Teach your child to call poison control, and get an adult involved right away. Make sure your child knows how to keep the bottle handy and give any information the dispatch needs.

The more information you give your child, the more prepared they are to handle the situation.

Something you need is stuck in a place you can't get to

Whether you are worried about a toy that has fallen where you can't reach it, or a pet that has climbed to where you can't reach it, get an adult and tell them you need help.

Children can get themselves into places they shouldn't be, or into situations that could be dangerous simply by following a pet or trying to reach a toy. Ensure your child knows that you are there to help, and stop him from going into places he shouldn't.

Something happens to your mom or dad when you are out in public

Accidents happen, and they can happen to the people we love. Just like when something happens and you are at home, teach your child who to call and what to do if you are in a situation that requires help when you are out in public.

Teach your child to call 911, and to go to the nearest store or sales associate for help, regardless of the situation you face.

You get separated from your group and have to do something you know you're not supposed to do to get back with them

It can be a tough call knowing when to make a decision on your own, and when you only have the basic rules to follow, this decision can be even harder.

For example:

If you have strict rules about crossing the street without an adult, but your child gets separated from you and must cross the street to reach you, he's going to have a tough time knowing what decision to make on his own.

When things like this happen, it's important that you teach him how to safely handle the situation, and alert a trusted adult to what's going on.

Again, if your child has a cell phone, have him call you or whoever he is with, and make sure he stays safe as he handles the situation.

You hurt yourself

Many children don't handle the sight of blood very well, and the thought of getting hurt and having to make a decision to handle it themselves can be frightening.

Teach your child where the first aid kit is, or if he's out in public how to choose a trusted adult to talk to.

Reassure your child that no matter what happened he's going to be ok, and he simply needs to remain calm, put a bandage on it if possible, and alert an adult.

No matter what lesson you are teaching your child, teach him to remain calm when handling a situation. As I said, it can be terrifying to a child to make a decision on his own, especially when he doesn't know what the right decision is.

But, if you take the time to show him a variety of situations, he's going to be prepared for any kind of situation that arises.

You see, it doesn't always matter how many scenarios you present your child with, if you teach him *how* to solve a problem, he'll know how to handle countless situations you didn't immediately address.

Use this time to build confidence in your child and show him that things are going to be fine, and give him the confidence he needs to handle situations himself. Though it's not that big a deal to us, the knowledge of how to handle a situation can make a world of difference to a child.

Good luck!

Conclusion

There you have it, everything you need to know to give your child the confidence they need to solve problems, and just what you need to teach your child to handle a variety of situations.

It can be hard knowing what kind of situations to address when you are teaching your child safety, and when you look over all the lessons in this book things can get overwhelming.

But, taking it slow is key to making it through, and showing your child bit by bit what to do will help the decisions stick for a long time.

I hope this book was able to inspire you to prepare your child for anything, and I hope you not only take the lessons in this book, but that you also add in more personalized lessons that address your own situation. No one knows the kind of life your child lives on a day to day basis better than you, and the more you can prepare your child for what could happen, the easier it's going to be for you.

Be patient, and be confident, and rest assured you have it handled. Your child is capable of learning so many things, and could surprise you with the answers he has when you first ask him how he would handle a situation.

Simply teach him why you want him to do things a certain way, and what to do when the unexpected happens, and you're going to prepare him in every way you are!

Now get out there and take on the world.

FREE BONUS REMINDER

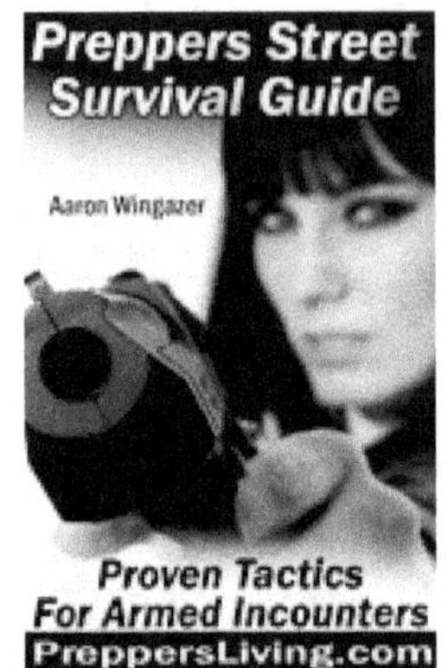

If you have not grabbed it yet, please go ahead and download your special bonus report *"Preppers Survival Guide. Proven Tactics For Armed Incounters!"*

Simply Click the Button Below

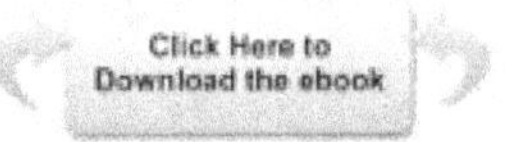

OR **Go to This Page**

http://preppersliving.com/free

BONUS #2: More Free & Discounted Books & Products

Do you want to receive more Free/Discounted Books or Products?

We have a mailing list where we send out our new Books or Products when they go free or with a discount on Amazon. Click on the link below to sign up for Free & Discount Book & Product Promotions.

=> Sign Up for Free & Discount Book & Product Promotions <=

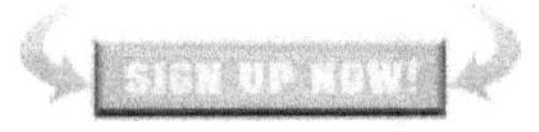

OR Go to this URL

http://zbit.ly/1WBb1Ek